DR. MICHAEL STERN

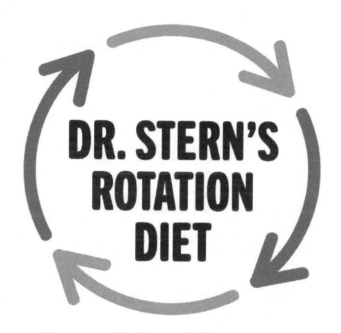

DR. STERN'S
ROTATION
DIET

Lose Fast. Lose Forever.

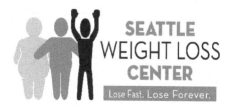

SEATTLE
WEIGHT LOSS
CENTER
Lose Fast. Lose Forever.

Published by

Seattle Weight Loss Center
PO Box 27383
Seattle, WA 98165
www.SeattleWeightLossCenter.org

ISBN 978-0-578-81690-6

Library of Congress Control Number: 2020951406

Designed and printed in the United States of America

I dedicate this book to my two siblings who died from complications of obesity, and to my three uncles who died from heart disease. All were very young.

I also dedicate it to all those inspirational quadriplegics who thrive despite tremendous challenges, particularly Jim Ryan, a Canadian pilot who inspired me to do all I can with the rest of my life.

CONTENTS

INTRODUCTION

If you're reading this, you know you need help. I knew *I* needed help. I was tooling around Chicagoland in my sporty Pontiac Bonneville on a beautiful day in the early sixties, the wind in my hair, The Beatles and The Four Tops on the radio, and I was angry. I pulled alongside a practice field to watch the players scrimmage in the afternoon sun.

I was an all-around athlete. You name it, I did it. In school, I focused on baseball, basketball, and football, pushing myself as hard as I could, striving to be the best of the best. And I was pretty good, but far from great, and certainly not good enough to compete with those players on that football field on that summer afternoon in the sixties.

But I knew I could be. One thing that I had in my corner was an ironclad work ethic. I may have lacked the natural talent that some players brought to the game, but I had the drive and the willingness—the *eagerness*—to put in the hours. If I wasn't born with it, I would simply have to outwork them.

So I did. I practiced in the early mornings and the late evenings, I built up my strength and endurance, I sharpened my skills, I ran in the park and threw balls and lifted weights while the other kids cruised along Lake Shore Drive or sat at home watching *Gunsmoke* or *Dragnet*. But no matter how hard I worked, I always came up short. I tried to convince myself that the problem was favoritism, or fate, or just plain bad luck. The real problem, though, was far simpler and it was something that I didn't want to have to deal with: I was overweight.

Sure, I could slug the ball, but I was slow around the bases. I could whip the pigskin fifty yards, but I was too slow to dodge a tackle. I could swish a basketball right through the hoop (and I'm short), but I couldn't weave down the court. Players who lacked my skill and brains ran circles around me. Simply put, there was no way for me to compete with the same speed and grace as the other players without losing some serious weight. So I put myself on a weight-loss diet.

It worked. I lost the weight in record time and lettered in all three sports—the only person in my class to do so. I even became the president of the lettermen's club.

I had done it. I become an excellent all-around amateur athlete; earned the admiration of faculty, friends, and girls; and was well on my way to a bright, happy future devoid of worry and trouble. Except for one thing.

The weight came back.

I thought I was done. I thought I had conquered my weight issues and that it would be smooth sailing from here on out. I couldn't have been more wrong. Like many, I spent a lot of time as a yo-yo dieter, achieving enormous results only to backslide and regain what I had lost. Some of this was due to slacking off with the discipline (something that nearly all of us are guilty of), but much of it was that, after a while, any given diet stopped being effective. Why this happens, and what to do about it, is one of the primary elements of my weight-loss program, *Dr. Stern's Rotation Diet*.

The sad truth is that our bodies are designed to gain weight, and keeping our natural biological tendencies in check is a never-ending battle (that's where the work ethic comes in). There is no silver bullet that guarantees lifelong success, especially as our bodies age and change, but I have found a method that works, and it will work for you. It enabled me, someone who is naturally inclined to be overweight, to be a top athlete; it enabled me to achieve and maintain my ideal weight range for periods of my life (when I stuck with it); and it enables me to control my weight today. That last part is significant. Here's why: In 1995 I was diagnosed with multiple sclerosis. My condition has grown progressively worse, to the point that I am a virtual quadriplegic (I have limited use of one arm). Workouts are impossible. The gym is off limits. My beloved sports are a thing of the past. Yet, through the method that I developed, I am *still* able to control my weight. Think about that the next time someone says they can't lose weight because they don't have the time to exercise or that their doctor told them not to because they have a bad back.

SO HOW DOES IT WORK?

Dr. Stern's Rotation Diet has four key components:

- Motivation
- Disciplined Endurance
- Diet
- Exercise

Unlike most weight-loss programs, however, I'm not here to convince you that any single weight-loss diet or any one fitness regimen is the key to success. On the contrary, Dr. Stern's Rotation Diet embraces variety, a characteristic that addresses a common fault with most weight-loss programs: *We get bored with them.* When we get bored, we lose discipline. When we lose discipline, we fail. My program will not bore you. Follow my program and you will not fail.

One quick note: The word *diet* simply refers to whatever food you habitually eat on a regular basis over a period of time. In popular usage, however, *diet* is often used interchangeably with *weight-loss program*. They are not the same thing. Keep this distinction in mind as we move through this book.

WHY AM I DOING THIS?

I spent most of my professional life as a urologist, a demanding field where, as with any other medical profession, a lack of attention to detail can be fatal. I brought this same level of scrutiny and rigor to my own weight loss efforts and, over the years, I've honed my theories through empirical observation and experience, contrasting my results with those of other, perhaps better-known programs with bigger advertising budgets. My passion led to the founding of the Seattle Weight Loss Center, a non-profit group that helps others discover what I've learned the hard way, providing free consultation and useful scientific information about the epidemic of obesity and how to combat it (Check us out at www.SeattleWeightLossCenter.org). Unlike many other programs, mine comes with no subscription fees and doesn't ask you to purchase special foods or meal packs. It *does* contain the key to long-term weight-loss success (which you'll learn by the end of the book), and it creates one pretty serious side effect: It generates enormous psychological benefits that will yield tremendous results in every area of your life. This side effect, and the ability to maintain your chosen weight range, will help you produce a lifetime of fitness and good health.

As I like to say, losing weight is simple, but it isn't easy. It isn't easy, but it's *worth it*. Is it worth it to you? Of course it is. A longer lifespan, better health, fewer doctor visits, better sleep, enhanced sex drive, making everyone jealous at the class reunion, and looking good in a bathing suit—all direct results of weight loss.

Lifetime weight maintenance requires a lifelong solution and that solution can be Dr. Stern's Rotation Diet. If you have the mental toughness to commit to it and see it through, you'll gain the confidence and power to tackle projects that you previously thought were beyond your reach: Get that job, earn that promotion, start that business, ask out that guy or gal, write that novel, climb that mountain (literally), and otherwise build a life that others only dream about. All of this and more can be yours, but only if you read the book and *take action* with the determination and resolve of someone who wants to take control and make tomorrow better than all of your yesterdays. Are you with me? Excellent. Turn the page.

DR. STERN'S WEIGHT-LOSS MAXIMS

Resolve now to do what it takes to lose weight and achieve your goals. Here are some ways to ensure your success.

Committing yourself to any program that can significantly alter your lifestyle, your health, and your longevity is serious business with serious implications. I'm not saying that you can't have fun with it; on the contrary, I hope you do. The more fun the better. But if we're to have any chance of success it's essential that we take it seriously on a fundamental level. Too many people embark upon weight-loss programs without thinking them through, without making the commitment, without preparing themselves to accept the occasional hardship or setback, and the result is always the same: *failure*. Success takes commitment, determination, mindfulness, and an unyielding belief in your ability to achieve the results you seek.

One important way to set the stage as we begin this journey is to establish a set of simple rules and concepts to keep in mind as we move forward. Read these maxims, think about them, be mindful of them, and keep them alive in your thoughts. They will provide a context for everything else that we'll do as we progress. Some of them are common sense, some may be new to you, others have implications that go far beyond weight loss, and all of them are key components of a successful program.

1. Our Bodies Are Designed to Gain Weight.

It's true. Evolution is a slow process. We have instant access to seemingly limitless quantities of food of every conceivable variety. Our cave-dwelling ancestors, on the other hand, had to work for every meal. Each bite of food could be their last. Food was scarce. Daily calorie intake was almost certainly well below requirements. And this is a situation that didn't improve for thousands of years. Only in the past few centuries has the Western World developed a system that supplies more food than our society can consume. That's great, food abundance is one of the hallmarks of a successful civilization. But here's the hitch: Our bodies still think it's the Stone Age. We are designed to pack on the pounds because we don't know when the next saber-toothed tiger or woolly mammoth will come down the pike and provide dinner. The extra body fat that we carry around could be the only thing that stands between life and an agonizing death

13

by starvation. Of course now, in the 21st century, we rarely have the opportunity to burn that body fat. It just sits there waiting for a famine that never arrives. There are ways to force your body to consume it (we'll get to that), but otherwise it's just a throwback to another time, and one that most of us would rather leave in the past.

Here's the most important thing to remember about this maxim, and I want you to remember this above all: Your body's natural tendency to gain weight is not your fault. You are *designed* to gain weight. Losing it, unless you're going to literally starve yourself (which I don't recommend), is hard. Keeping it off is harder. It takes work. So if things go backward a little, don't be too hard on yourself. Don't beat yourself up about it. But don't use it as an excuse, either. Just remind yourself that it's just your body doing what it's supposed to do, regroup, and move on. Your mind is stronger than your body. Use it.

2. You Are Always on a Diet

The question is, what kind of diet are you on? Are you on the random-food diet? The whatever's-put-in-front-of-me diet? The Doritos-and-beer diet? Maybe you're mindful and you try to stick to healthy, low-carb, low-fat foods. Maybe you try to be reasonable and eat all things in moderation. Or maybe you just eat and don't give your diet any thought at all. Regardless of what you eat, and regardless of whether or not you give it any thought, you are still on a diet every single day of your life.

The question is, as I said at the beginning, *what kind of diet are you on?* Whatever your eating habits may be, your diet is guaranteed to fall into one of three categories:

- A weight-gaining diet (WGD)
- A weight-maintenance (or weight-neutral) diet (WND)
- A weight-loss diet (WLD)

If, like many people, you don't give a great deal of thought to what you eat, the challenge is to start thinking about your diet as, yes, a *diet*. It's the first step in examining your habits so you can bring them in line with your goals. Curious about where your diet falls? Check the scale every morning and you'll find out. Which brings us to the next maxim.

3. It's a Lifelong Commitment

You don't adopt a fitness program for three months and then expect to reap the benefits for the rest of your life. Lasting benefits require a lasting commitment. Be faithful to your fitness program and your fitness program will be faithful to you.

The same applies to your weight-loss and weight-maintenance programs. You can't expect to adopt a regimen, achieve your goal, and then abandon it without also abandoning everything that you've gained. Stick with the program without fail and let it do its work.

4. Check the Scale Every Day

Scales are cheap. They're easy to use. You don't have to hook them up to the web (although you can if you want to). Get one and check your weight every day. Don't obsess over it. Don't turn it into a chore or a trial or a reason to get down on yourself if you aren't making progress. It's simply a matter of keeping track of what's going on with your body and noticing the subtle changes that occur when we alter our behaviors.

We see ourselves every day in the mirror. We notice a new wrinkle or a new gray hair. We pay attention when our car makes an unwelcome new sound. But weight creeps up on us. We don't realize how much it changes on a day-to-day basis unless we make a point to do so. And as important as general awareness is (and it *is* important), just like the noises your car makes, changes in your weight could be an early warning sign alerting you to potential trouble ahead. Buy a scale and use it.

5. Eat Fewer Calories and Expend More Energy

Calories are the fuel that keeps your body running. They're like gasoline to a car, except your car doesn't store unused gasoline around its fenders. That's why it's important that we learn to manage our intake and expenditure of calories. It's simple math, like a story problem you figure out with your body, although the numbers may be a little soft. You can count calories, but the amount of activity required to burn them depends upon how your body is wired up. Only you, through some intelligent experimentation, can figure that out, but one thing is certain: If you eat lower-calorie foods, or reduce your overall consumption, and increase your level of activity, your net caloric intake will diminish. It's a sure thing. Eat one less snack; walk one more mile. Repeat.

6. It's Movement, not Exercise

You'll notice that, until now, I have not used the E-word. *Exercise* sounds too much like work. *Movement* does not. Every time you move your body you will burn calories. It's impossible to do otherwise. Therefore, seek to move.

Some of us are gym rats and enjoy working out, but most of us would rather relax in the La-Z-Boy and watch the tube. Those of us who fall into the latter category aren't enticed by elliptical machines and free weights. But walking around the block doesn't sound too bad, right? How about standing for a while and shifting your weight from side to side instead of spending the evening in the recliner? Try picking a parking space that isn't the closest one to the door, take the stairs instead of the elevator, squeeze a stress ball while you bang away on your laptop, and dance around like a fool when no one is home. Or do it out in public. You'll burn calories either way.

The bottom line is this: Don't take the easiest option. Choose to walk ten steps instead of five. Choose to *move*.

7. Eating Saps Energy

After every Thanksgiving feast we spend a few hours struggling to keep our eyes open as a collective drowsiness settles over the family. We've been told that this happens because turkey contains a drowsiness-inducing amino acid called *tryptophan*. It's true that tryptophan can make you sleepy, and it's also true that turkey has some of nature's sleeping pill tucked away inside. However, as great as all of this sounds, the tryptophan in the turkey has nothing to do with our evening Thanksgiving nap. Turkey simply doesn't contain enough of it to make an impact.

What *does* make us sleepy is eating a high volume of food in a short amount of time. After the turkey and the stuffing and the mashed potatoes and the corn and whatever else you have room for, your body has to take all of that mass and do something with it. This is where digestion comes in, one of those out-of-sight-out-of-mind functions that your body does all the time without you having to worry about it. When you eat a large meal your body goes into overdrive trying to manage it. "But doesn't that burn calories?" you ask. Yes, it does, but not as many as you just ate. Eat smaller meals. Your body will handle the food more efficiently, it'll be easier to lose weight, and you won't feel that post-supper drag. And no, I'm not saying that you shouldn't eat Thanksgiving dinner. Just remember that we only do it once a year.

8. Follow the Money

Popular weight-loss programs are often less about helping you lose weight than they are about making someone else wealthy. I'm not mentioning any names, and I'm not saying that these programs lack value. By and large, they work. But they're designed to lock you into a system that requires endless monthly fees or ongoing purchases of branded foods designed exclusively for that program. If one of these paid programs is attractive to you, examine how it works and see if you can duplicate what they do without having to establish a perpetual bank transfer. There are plenty of good, proven programs that cost virtually nothing. And yes, I know you had to pay for this book, but I won't charge you a monthly fee to read it.

9. Motivate Yourself

Why do most weight-loss programs fail? It usually isn't because there's something wrong with the program. It's because we lose our motivation and slack off until we're right back where we were before we started. The typical New Year's resolution of *I want to lose weight* is rarely enough to get you to your goal. *I want to lose weight* isn't a good enough reason to keep the lid on that pint of Ben and Jerry's ice cream that mocks you from the freezer. There's a point where an ambiguous desire to lose weight can no longer resist the temptations of the snack aisle and the lure of laziness.

Strong motivation is *essential*. It's the single most important component of any successful weight-loss program. Ask yourself why you want to lose weight. Drill down. Be specific. Make it personal and express it in the first person. If the New Year's resolution doesn't do the trick, maybe "I'd like to meet my grandchildren" will. Figure out why you *really* want to lose weight. Repeat it to yourself first thing in the morning, at night just before bed, and at regular intervals throughout the day. Post reminders around the house and in the car (as silly as that sounds, it can be extremely effective). Above all, be clear with yourself about your reasons and never lose touch with them. If your motivation vanishes, so does your dieting program and all of the benefits that come with it.

10. MEA: Motivation, Education, Association

Take your motivation and augment it with knowledge and companionship. Learn all you can about how your body works, how it's affected by what you eat, and how changing your daily behaviors impacts your weight, your fitness, your mood, and your overall well-being. Knowledge is power and the more you know the better you'll be able to make adjustments and course corrections when necessary.

Associate with like-minded individuals and find one who can be your accountability partner. Make sure it's someone who understands what you're trying to do and will stand by you and support you even when things get tough; someone who isn't afraid to point out when you're dropping the ball, who will give you a shove when you're stuck, and who will tell you to snap out of it when you make excuses. Choose carefully. Your accountability partner can be instrumental in helping you achieve your goals, and might even become a friend for life.

11. Cut Your Portions in Half

Do it right now. You don't even have to wait until you've finished the book. However much you usually cook, cut it in half. However much you usually eat, eat half. If you go out to eat, ask the server to box up half your meal right at the outset (this will also get you two meals for the price of one).

Halving your serving sizes is the easiest way to begin any long-term weight-loss program. It helps ease you into the changes to come, and it acclimates your body to a lower food intake (which is good because, like most people, you've probably been eating too much anyway).

12. Remove Unhealthy Foods From the Premises

Unhealthy foods include junk foods and *any other* foods that aren't a part of your current weight-loss or dietary regimen. Simply having these foods around the house and within your reach will tempt you to indulge in recreational eating that subverts your weight-loss efforts. Get rid of them.

13. Get Busy!

Some people want to lose weight. Some people just like to dream about it. Be a doer, not a dreamer. You can do it, but it requires you to take action and make it happen. Reading this book is only the first step. It's time to get busy. Resolve now to do what it takes to lose that weight and achieve your goals. Your new life is within your grasp. You only have to reach out and take it.

One More Piece of Good Advice: Keep a journal. Record your weight every day and monitor your progress. You can even plot it on a graph if you like. Also record your impressions of the various diets that you'll try as part of Dr. Stern's Rotation Diet. How well do the diets work? Which ones do you like? What tips and tricks have you learned? How does each diet make you feel, both physically and mentally? The simple act of writing things down will help keep you engaged with your dieting and will provide a handy reference work in the future.

Chapter 1

WHAT'S OUT THERE AND WHY YOU SHOULD KNOW

There is a broad spectrum of weight-loss programs available, but they fall within common categories. Understanding them will help you make intelligent decisions in the future.

When I was younger and exploring the many weight-loss programs that were available, I often took a bit of a contrarian attitude. In the 1970s, when I was still an athlete, I was in a weight-loss group (a big one with a name you would recognize) with people who mostly spent their days at home leading sedentary lives. I, on the other hand, was running three to six miles a day. I couldn't relate to the group and the group couldn't relate to me. When I suggested that they might want to get outside and move around a little I was admonished for being too outspoken and asked to leave.

Later, I joined another group (again, a big one with a name you would recognize). This one mandated ongoing purchases of their branded food products, a requirement that I rebelled against (and yes, I joined voluntarily, but I just can't help but push back; it's in my nature). When I lost more weight than my advisor, and did it largely without eating the company's foods, it didn't make anyone very happy. When I challenged my advisor to a weight-loss contest I was promptly asked to leave once again. After all, what was the point of me being around if I wasn't making money for the company by buying their stuff?

Then I attended a weight-loss clinic in Panama where I was allowed only one type of fruit per meal, with no mixing or matching. It was bad news for me when I decided to throw some melon in with my banana. Oh, well. At least the beaches were nice.

These experiences, and many others, weren't the wastes of time that they may appear to be. Far from it. They opened my eyes to the endless variety of weight-loss programs that are available, and the fact that, for all of that variety, there are only so many ways to lose weight. In fact, when you get right down to it, there's really only one: Consume fewer calories than your body uses to convert into energy. This forces you to tap into your fat reserves and, *voilà*, you lose weight. It's as simple as that. Weight loss is an imprecise enterprise, however, and while it all boils down to the same thing, there are any number of ways to approach it.

Dr. Stern's Rotation Diet embraces variety, and not just of food types. The keystone of my program is *dietary rotation.* Adopt one diet, follow it for a while, let it do its work, and then consciously and carefully switch to another. We'll go into more detail later, but for now it's important to know that the rotation method accomplishes two primary objectives. The first is that rotation overcomes your body's natural inclination to adapt to circumstances. Any number of diets are effective in the short term, but when your body figures out what you're up to it will work hard to undermine your goals. Remember, *your body wants to store fat* which, unless you're a body builder, is how most of us gain weight. Your body will find ways to work around your weight-loss schemes. Rotate your diet and keep your body on its toes.

The second objective is this: If your body's natural inclination is to store fat, your *mind's* natural inclination is to get bored. Even the most fascinating pastime eventually becomes tedious. Your diet is no exception, and when you get bored with your diet you can probably kiss your weight-loss efforts goodbye. Rotation addresses this. Keep your diet new and you'll keep your mind engaged.

BREAKING IT DOWN

Dietary rotation isn't as simple as rolling dice or flipping coins. Doing it intelligently requires some knowledge of the broad categories of diets that are available, how they work, how they differ from one another, and what distinguishes some of the popular programs. Bear in mind that every type of diet has its champions and detractors; for any given example, there are those who'll say it works like a charm and others who'll say it's a load of hooey. The truth is that, while there might be a little hooey in any specific diet, all of these diets *work*. Let me say that again: THEY ALL WORK, and they can all be adopted as weight-loss programs if you follow them faithfully. I'll make no effort to explain *everything* that's out there and available—that would be a whole book in itself—but it's enough to know that most diets fall into one of the following categories:

- Calorie Counting
- Common Sense/Mindfulness
- Ideology
- Low Carb
- Low Fat
- Meal Replacement
- Fasting

To help you navigate this landscape, and to help you make decisions as we move further along this journey, let's take a quick look at the major categories of diets and a few examples of popular programs in each.

CALORIE-COUNTING DIETS

Calorie-counting diets drill right down to the ultimate foundation of every diet: the creation of a calorie deficit. Burn more calories than you consume and you will lose weight. By keeping track of your caloric intake, running it through a height-and-weight formula, and making some assumptions about your daily activity levels, a calorie-counting diet attempts to approximate a diet that will keep you on a calorie deficit without forcing you to go hungry. Like all diets, it's imprecise. Modern food labeling helps, but things can get pretty complicated when you have to count the calories in a scratch-cooked meal.

Here are a couple of examples of calorie-counting diets:

WW (Weight Watchers): Weight Watchers has shortened its name to WW which, despite its brevity, has twice as many syllables as the old one. Rest assured that, with tweaks and refinements, it's still the same system that's been around for years. It uses calorie counting—along with a host of other considerations, like the presence of saturated fats and processed sugars—to assign a point system to foods. A counselor helps you assign a point budget that tells you how much of which types of foods you can eat and still lose weight. One great benefit of WW is that no foods are off limits as long as they fit within your daily point budget. You can eat anything. WW is a subscription system with a proprietary point-counter app that requires monthly fees. It's specifically designed for gradual, long-term weight loss. Specialized food products are available, but they aren't required by the program.

For obvious reasons, subscription-based programs aren't the best choices for rotation diets, but WW is too big and popular to go unmentioned.

Simple Calorie Counting: This is the way we used to do it: Buy a calorie-counting book, check your height and weight against the table in the first few pages, look up your recommended daily calorie budget, use the book's calorie charts for every type of food imaginable, and plan your meals accordingly. In other words, it's a stripped-down, less sophisticated version of WW without the fees. In the old days you could get a little mechanical pocket device to keep track of your intake. Nowadays there's an app for that.

One great benefit to this type of diet is that it really makes you pay attention to what you eat. It forces you to be aware of, and account for, every single snack. That, in itself, is a major step forward for many of us.

COMMON-SENSE/MINDFULNESS DIETS

While calorie counting forces us to be aware of what we eat, common sense diets are *explicitly* about dietary awareness: *Be aware of what you eat.* We all have a pretty good idea of what constitutes a healthy diet: more fruits and vegetables, less cake and ice cream, and eat nothing in excess. These programs take that concept and apply some structure and discipline to help keep you on track.

Here are some examples:

Mediterranean Diet: If you like seafood, this one is for you. Heavy on fish, nuts, and grains at the expense of sugar and processed meats, this program approximates the traditional diets of Greece, Italy, and the French Riviera, all areas famous for outstanding cuisine and for the overall good health and longevity of their residents. Bonus inducement: Red wine is a bona fide component of the Mediterranean diet, so drink up if you're so inclined.

Paleo Diet: This diet assumes that we should confine ourselves to the foods that our bodies are evolutionarily equipped to handle (mostly plants, nuts, and lean meats) and avoid those that we are not (processed foods, sugars, and Cheetos). The paleo diet has more than its share of detractors, with some saying that it is deficient in calcium and proteins, but as with any other diet, using it on a rotational basis with other programs will mitigate any potential issues.

Jenny Craig: Like WW, Jenny Craig is a subscription program that focuses on simple, healthy eating. Clients are encouraged to adopt a diet built on foods provided by the company—for a fee, of course—thereby relieving you of the work of having to figure these things out for yourself (which, of course, means that while this may be a common-sense diet, it isn't really a *mindfulness* diet).

Also like WW, Jenny Craig has a robust promotional machine that keeps it in the spotlight; and like any other subscription-based program, it's not a great choice for a rotation diet.

IDEOLOGICAL DIETS

Ideological diets are primarily driven by philosophy or ethos, chief among them the concept that we ought not to eat other animals. It also illustrates how some diet categories overlap (you could make the case for the paleo diet being an ideological diet). But there is one ideological diet that looms above them all.

Vegetarian/Vegan Diet: There's a spectrum here, from those who think that fish don't count as animals, to those who won't eat meat but think it's okay to use animal products (like eggs and milk), to those who advocate an entirely plant-based diet that excludes anything that comes from a creature with a heartbeat. Those on the vegetarian end of the spectrum are more likely to be driven by the perceived health benefits, while those on the vegan (100% plant) end are more likely to be driven by ideology. The biggest issue with most of these diets is that they omit types of food that omnivores are explicitly designed to consume, leaving us wanting for important nutritional components for which we otherwise have to compensate. In other words, people are *supposed* to eat meat and, when we don't, we have to address its absence. These diets can help you lose weight, just make sure to take some supplements when you're on one of them.

LOW-CARB DIETS

Low-carbohydrate diets have been pretty fashionable over the last fifteen years or so. Here's a simple explanation of how they work: Carbohydrates are your body's primary energy source. During digestion, carbs are converted into sugars which are then injected into your bloodstream. Rising blood-sugar levels trigger a corresponding increase in insulin production. Insulin helps transfer blood sugar to cells where some of it is stored as fat.

When you slash your carb consumption you also slash your insulin production. Diminished insulin levels cause your body to burn stored fat in a process called *ketosis*. When your body is in a state of ketosis you can lose weight quickly. If you can sacrifice bread and potatoes, a low-carb diet can help you achieve rapid weight loss.

The first diet that I tried, and the one that provided great results when I was young, was the Stillman Diet, developed by Dr. Irwin Maxwell Stillman in 1967. While the Stillman Diet has gone by the wayside, many of Dr. Stillman's theories live on in today's low-carb diets, especially the first example in this list:

Atkins Diet: Named after its developer, Dr. Robert Atkins, this diet has been enduringly popular since the early 1970s and it's still going strong today. The reasons are twofold: It can make a fast and obvious difference in your body weight, and it allows you to eat high-fat foods (because insulin production is triggered by carbs, not fats). The Atkins Diet is high on proteins, so all the meats are on the menu: beef, pork, chicken, seafood, you name it. Carbs, on the other hand, are not, and we're not just talking about the usual suspects of breads and potatoes. Fruits are also strongly discouraged. In short, if you enjoy eating guilt-free cheeseburgers, this diet is an excellent choice. Just make sure you skip the bun.

A final note: Some complain that Atkins is great in the short term, but doesn't work well for maintaining your target weight. Nonetheless, fast-acting diets can be great choices for rotation diets, so keep this one in mind.

Keto Diet: Sort of an amplified Atkins Diet, the keto diet cuts carbs down to the bone (about five percent of daily intake) and ramps up the proteins and, especially, the fats. Unlike Atkins, which aims to put you back on something that resembles a normal diet after your weight loss is accomplished, the keto diet is intended to be permanent.

South Beach Diet: This diet addresses what its designers saw as a heart-health deficiency in existing low-carb diets like Atkins. South Beach discourages high-fat proteins (which Atkins allows), and permits what it calls "good carbs," like fruits and whole grains (which are verboten under Atkins). Since it's essentially a somewhat re-engineered version of the Atkins Diet, this one might be a good transitional diet in a rotational plan.

LOW-FAT DIETS

Possibly the granddaddy of all weight-loss programs, a low-fat diet pretty much speaks for itself and can be as basic and simple as trimming the fat from your steak. In fact, the whole concept of "low fat" has so permeated our society that most of us probably don't realize that there was a time when we not only didn't trim the fat rinds from our meats, we made a point of *eating* them. You'd be hard pressed to find anyone doing that now.

Here's an example of a low-fat diet:

Pritiken Diet: This diet is low-fat all the way, encouraging white meats over red, heavy consumption of fruits and vegetables, limiting alcohol, and emphasizing high-fiber foods (which have their own way of removing weight from your body). One criticism of this diet has been that, while effective, people get bored with it because of the heavy limitations on food choice.

Which, of course, makes it a perfect diet for a rotational program.

MEAL-REPLACEMENT DIETS

Meal-replacement diets substitute a prepared food of some kind, often a bar or a shake, for one or more traditional meals. The substitutes, which are created by scientists and dietitians (hopefully), are designed to fulfill your nutritional requirements, satisfy your hunger, and reduce your calorie load. Not all meal-substitution diets work the same way. Some ask you to use the product exclusively; others suggest using them to replace only one or two of your traditional three meals. And note that they are *products*. While you may be able to whip up your own substitutions, most such diets require spending money on prepared packages.

OPTIFAST: Yes, they write it in all caps, and it's a proven program that works. OPTIFAST is a medically supervised program that substitutes 100% of your meals with proprietary meal-replacement products for an active weight-loss period of twelve to sixteen weeks. Then, for four to six weeks, you transition back to a diet of traditional foodstuffs, albeit one that follows an OPTIFAST-approved plan. After the transition is complete, it's up to you to stay the course. Remember that, unlike most other diets, OPTIFAST requires medical supervision and it does cost money. On the other hand, unlike many other subscription plans, the goal of OPTIFAST is to help you achieve weight loss, set you up for ongoing success, and then wean you off of their products and services.

SlimFast: Available over the counter and designed to replace a single meal, not your entire diet, SlimFast has a heavy protein content and lots of fiber—the latter helps keep the hunger pangs away. This is a sound alternative to a complete meal, and a good complement to a broader weight-loss program.

There are other meal-replacement products available, but steer yourself toward those that have a track record. Don't let yourself be the guinea pig for the latest thing to hit the market.

ONE FINAL DIET

This one is in a class by itself, and it's not one that you can do for the long haul: *fasting*. It's not fun, but putting yourself on a water-only diet for a couple of days is entirely doable and it can produce remarkable results. It's how I jump-started my own weight loss decades ago and I recommend it as a starting point, especially if your weight-loss goals are significant. Fast for two days, then put yourself on a diet.

Even a partial fast can be effective: Confine your consumption period to a six-to-eight-hour window and fast for the remainder of the day. This is an excellent option for those who would like to experience some of the benefits of fasting without the attendant discomfort. It's also a good alternative for those who would like to fast during the work week when it makes sense to keep a little food on your stomach to stave off distraction. Whichever path you choose, after a fast your new diet, and its rules, will seem less restrictive, you will savor every bite, and you will be well on your way to a healthy and sustainable lifestyle.

IMPORTANT NOTE: Fasting for longer periods of time (more than two days) is not a project for amateurs, but it can be done safely at a destination inpatient clinic such as TrueNorth Health Center in Santa Rosa, California, where I spent two years on staff.

Summing it up . . .

- There is really only one way to lose weight: Consume fewer calories than your body uses to convert into energy.

- All of these diets work and can be adapted into weight-loss programs.

- Dr. Stern's Rotation Diet is a more effective method than following one diet exclusively.

- Weight-loss diets fall into one of seven general categories: calorie counting, common sense/mindfulness, ideology, low carb, low fat, and meal replacement, fasting.

- Each diet uses a different method to achieve weight loss.

Chapter 2

READY TO LAUNCH: WHAT WORKS AND WHAT DOESN'T

Common misconceptions can hinder your progress. Here's what you need to know about what to embrace and what to ignore.

If losing weight were easy, no one would need to lose weight. It's a challenge. It takes work and effort and dedication. It takes focus. And it's hard enough without wasting your time (and sometimes your money) on programs that don't work well or, sometimes, don't work at all. What works and what doesn't is often a matter of common sense, but some things are more obvious than others. I know I said that all diets work, but some defy common sense. A strictly celery diet isn't healthy; don't try it. Here's a quick survey of things to look out for when evaluating weight-loss programs.

WHAT DOESN'T WORK

Anything that says you don't have to work. As I said, weight loss requires effort, and it often requires sacrifice. Even if it's as simple as being mindful of what you eat, or swearing off your ice cream habit, you still have to do *something*. And taking a magic pill that was advertised on a late-night infomercial doesn't count. Anything that sounds too good to be true probably is, and anyone who promises a medical miracle that makes you shed pounds while lounging on the couch is selling you 21st century snake oil. Don't buy it.

Fad Diets. Fad diets come and go so quickly they barely even register in our memories: The iceberg-lettuce diet, the Italian meatball diet, the twelve-tiny-meals diet, the antipasto diet, the un-cooked-flour diet, you name it. I made those diets up, but they're not too far off the mark. Here are some real ones (and I've tried them): the grapefruit diet, the cabbage-soup diet, and the peanut-butter-and-banana diet. In addition to being generally ineffective, fad diets often ignore basic nutritional concepts and can be hazardous. "But Dr. Stern," you ask, "how do I know if a new diet is a *fad* diet?" Good question. Here are two ways to tell:

1). It defies common sense. An iceberg-lettuce diet sounds like a bad idea because it *is* a bad idea, and you know that instinctively without needing an expert's guidance. If something seems wrong, don't let yourself be convinced otherwise.

2). It has no history. Diets that have endured the test of time are not fad diets. They're still around because they work. Fad diets, by definition, peak quickly and then disappear, usually because they are founded on faulty principles. A diet with a track record of success is one that's been around a while, so when it's time to choose, go with one that has some history. Atkins, Pritikin, South Beach, et al., are tried and true, well-documented, and definitely not fads. Go with diets like these and avoid disappointment.

Using exercise as a weight-loss program. I am *not* telling you to avoid the gym! Exercise is great (remember, I prefer to call it *movement*), but the key to weight loss is calorie control. You can tone your muscles, stay fit, and increase your cardiopulmonary endurance—all laudable goals—but unless you also control your diet, significant weight loss is unlikely to occur through movement alone.

Power bars and protein shakes. There's nothing wrong with using these to help out, but some of us rely on them as if they are panaceas and valid replacements for every meal. They are not and, when overused, they can actually cause you to gain weight. Stick to real food and you'll be far better off.

Dieting for superficial reasons. This is the biggest problem of all, and it's one we discussed briefly in the *Maxims* chapter. Go read that again because it bears repeating (and this isn't the last time I'll bring it up): Without the right motivation, without a compelling and driving purpose, you will fail. I don't say this to discourage you; I say it because now, at the beginning of your journey, is the time to tap into and harness that wellspring of resolve that will carry you through the challenging times ahead.

WHAT WORKS

What works is a program of proven weight-loss theories, used in rotation, applied with uncompromising discipline. Dr. Stern's Rotation Diet combines diets from a series of successful weight-loss programs in rotation to create synergy among several different diets. Just as different antibiotics are combined to cure more infections, and chemotherapy drugs are combined to get better results in treating cancer, so Dr. Stern's rotation diet. combines differing principles of weight loss to bring you the best of all of them. It allows you to reap the benefits of a host of different methods instead of settling for a narrower benefit provided by only one. And that's what we'll talk about in the next chapter.

Summing it up . . .

- **Common misconceptions about weight loss can hinder your progress.**
- **Any program that says *you* don't have to work will not work.**
- **Fad diets often do not work.**
- **Using exercise alone to lose weight does not work.**
- **Using power bars and protein shakes exclusively can result in weight gain.**
- **Successful weight loss relies upon strong motivation.**
- **The most successful program combines proven weight-loss theories, used in rotation, and applied with uncompromising discipline.**

Chapter 3

GETTING STARTED: THE BEST QUICK WEIGHT-LOSS PROGRAM

A short water-only fast can jump start your weight loss and pave the way for long-term success.

As I said at the beginning, if you're reading this book you know you need help. Oftentimes, we only admit we need help when we've gained enough weight that we can no longer

59

overlook it. If this describes you, one of the best ways to jump-start your weight-loss program and initiate Dr. Stern's Rotation Diet is with a water-only fast. Hospitals regularly put patients on intravenous sugar-water or salt-water diets as a means of promoting healing after gallbladder, pancreatic, or bowel diseases, and just prior to surgery (this practice is known as NPO, which is an abbreviation for *nil per os*, which is Latin for *nothing by mouth*—doctors like to use Latin). Start with a water-only fast and then move into a transitional mode toward the rotation diet (which we'll talk more about soon).

Your body needs fuel all the time, whether you're eating or not. Fasting forces your body to burn its stored fat—it literally has no choice—triggering rapid weight reduction. As you might imagine, fasting isn't always a pleasant experience. The benefits are real, though, and there are ways to make it at least tolerable.

TIPS FOR (ALMOST) PAINLESS FASTING

Ease Into it. Don't go off food cold-turkey if you have no experience with this sort of thing. Prepare yourself by cutting back gradually so that you aren't instantly switching from "eat whatever I want" to "eat nothing but water." Skip one meal a day, then skip two, and when you *do* eat, eat less than you typically would (you aren't doing yourself any favors if you eat one meal a day and overdo it). Reduce your sugars and carbs. Get your body used to making do with less before you pull the rug out from under it.

Prepare Your Mind. Too often, we overlook the psychological aspects of dieting and weight loss. If you want to shed some pounds, your mind is more important than your mouth. We'll discuss this at length in a later chapter, but for now just know that it's essential to mentally prepare yourself for some discomfort and inconvenience. If you know to expect it, and you've steeled yourself for the challenge, you'll find that the experience is 100% easier to endure than if you just stumbled into it as if nothing unusual was about to happen.

Remind yourself of why you're doing it. Remind yourself of the benefits that await on the other side of your fast. Remind yourself that the discomfort is temporary, that you've been through much worse, and that you'll only be doing it for a short time.

Above all, remind yourself that you *will succeed*, and that success requires work, a few sacrifices along the way, and keeping yourself motivated. Millions of people have done it before you. You can do it, too.

MAKE SURE IT'S OKAY. Water fasting should not be done if you have any significant medical problems such as diabetes, kidney disease, or liver disease, without first consulting your healthcare provider. Also, check any medications that you're taking and ensure that they aren't affected by food intake. And lastly, even if you have no medical issues, never fast for more than two days unless you are under medical supervision.

HOW IS IT DONE?

Here are two quick weight-loss programs, the first of which begins with a short fast.

The Quickest Weight-Loss Program: This is a supercharged method that promises the fastest results. Important note: Do not exercise during water-only fasts. Save it for later.

1. Begin with two days of water-only fasting. One common side-effect of fasting is headache (in fact, headache is a universal symptom; just about any disruption or malady can give you a headache). A pinch of salt added to your

water will help keep headaches at bay and will also help combat the mental fog that often accompanies an empty stomach. Acid reflux is another common side effect. A couple tablespoons of lemon juice in your water will help keep that under control and make your fast as tolerable as possible.

If nausea is an issue, try adding two ounces of cranberry juice, lemon drops, or watermelon juice to sixteen ounces of water and alternate with two ounces of vegetable or chicken both with every sixteen ounces of water. You can drink these hot or cold.

Arrange your fasting period so that you are free to do as little as possible. Maximize sleep and minimize movement. Relax. Snooze. Meditate. If you must do something, try engaging in a guilt-free binge of your favorite TV show. I give you permission. The bottom line is do *not* do any strenuous work or exercise.

2. After your 48-hour water fast, transition to four days of a supplemental-liquid program. You'll still be forgoing solid foods (sorry, but just think of how much you'll have to look forward to when you're done!), but three times a day you can treat yourself to a liquid Carnation Instant Breakfast mixed with nonfat skim milk (follow manufacturer's instructions). After three days of nothing but water, you'll appreciate the simple pleasures of flavored milk more than you'd ever thought possible.

3. Next, transition to a seven-day ketogenic diet. After seven days of a liquid diet your body will be burning its stored fat, which is exactly the goal. Now that

you've reached it, you can reintroduce some solid ketogenic-friendly foods that will allow your body to ramp up its nutrient intake, continue your fat-burning course, and satisfy your pent-up cravings for "real" food. Limit your diet to eggs, milk, cottage cheese, cheddar cheese, cream cheese, turkey, beef, pork, chicken, fish, steamed vegetables (especially broccoli and cauliflower), raw vegetables (especially lettuce, cucumber, and tomatoes), and a daily dose of a half-cup of Brazil nuts, pecans, or walnuts. Important: resist the urge to gorge yourself on your first meal after your fast. Doing so could result in indigestion, headaches (again), and other nasty side effects. Your body has grown accustomed to a lack of solid food. Ease back into it with half-portions or less (As a rule, you should always cut the recommended portion on food packaging by fifty percent). After a day or two you can begin to eat normal portions again.

WATER IN AND WATER OUT

Since you're about to embark on a water-only fast, now is a good time to take a small detour: How much water should you drink? This is one of the questions I'm most commonly asked, and I'm shocked by some of the answers I hear in the media, many of which are inadequate at best and dangerous at worst.

We are often led to believe that we should drink as much as we can. I once had a patient who wondered why she urinated so frequently. She produced four liters of urine a day (which is way too much). I reduced her water intake and cured her problem.

But it isn't simply a matter making too many trips to the bathroom. In 2002, a marathon runner in Boston died of hyponatraemia caused by excessive water consumption. In 2007, a Los Angeles radio station held a contest to see who could drink the most water. The second-place winner died of acute water toxicity. In short, you *can* drink too much water.

What are the variables that affect how much water you *should* drink? Some people recommend eight eight-ounce glasses a day (that's sixty-four ounces for the non-math people), but this common advice is an oversimplification of an issue that is very dependent on other factors. Here's what to keep in mind when determining appropriate water intake:

1. Current state of hydration
2. Current daily food intake
3. Ambient temperature and humility
4. Physical activity

5. Level of perspiration
6. Kidney function if normal

So how do we determine if our water intake is healthy? By measuring what comes out when our body is done with it. I recommend measuring your urinary output for a seventy-two hours (three days) to get a baseline. Assuming a normal renal function, it's recommended that you have 2,000 to 2,500 milliliters (ml) every twenty-four hours, or approximately 100 ml per hour. If your output is under 2,000 ml or over 3,000 ml you are either drinking too little or too much. If your food intake is stable, then you know if you have a diet which is water neutral or water dense or devoid of water. If your diet is high in water-dense foods like watermelon, iceberg lettuce, celery, and other foods that are filled with natural water, you won't need to drink as much. On the other hand, if your diet that is filled with foods low in water, such as animal products, grains, bread, and pasta you'll have to drink more.

Keep this in mind as you embark on your water-only fast. Keep track of your urinary output. It shouldn't change dramatically. Oh, and one more thing: The easiest way to avoid the agony of kidney stones (and believe me, they hurt) is to maintain a healthy water intake and a urinary output of at least 2,000 ml a day.

Now let's get back to the weight-loss programs.

The Quick (but not the Quickest) Weight-Loss Program: This is an easier program for those who aren't up to the challenge of a fast, or who may have medical conditions that contraindicate fasting.

1. Go on a two-week, high-carbohydrate, largely plant-based program of vegetables, eggs, and dairy. Here's what three typical meals might look like:

   Breakfast: Two tablespoons of cottage cheese, two soft-boiled eggs, coffee (with

2% milk if you like, but no sugar), and three Brazil nuts or walnuts.

Lunch: Lettuce, tomato, and cucumber salad with no dressing; steamed broccoli, cauliflower, and carrots; and one stalk of celery with peanut butter.

Supper: One bowl of white or brown rice mixed with onion, bell pepper, carrots, and two ounces of broiled chicken or turkey.

Snacks: Plain air-popped popcorn, no butter or salt.

2. Alternate this high-carb diet: eggs, milk, cottage cheese, cheddar cheese, cream cheese, turkey, beef, pork, chicken, fish, steamed vegetables (especially broccoli and cauliflower), raw vegetables (especially lettuce, cucumber, and tomatoes), and a daily dose of a half-cup of Brazil nuts, pecans, or walnuts. Determine which diet, high-carb or ketogenic, results in the most significant weight loss. Our bodies

are all different and what works wonders for one person may be less effective for another.

Once you've gone through one of the above rapid-reduction diets you may be ready to transition into Dr. Stern's Rotation Diet, designed to keep you on an even keel and maintain a weight within your chosen healthy range. So take a breather, then come back here and we'll continue into the heart of what Dr. Stern's Rotation Diet is all about.

Summing it up . . .

- One of the best ways to jump start a weight-loss program is with a two-day water-only fast.

- Fasting forces your body to tap into its fat reserves.

- Ease into fasting, and prepare your mind for the task.

- Ensure that there are no medical issues that could prevent you from fasting safely.

- Never fast for more than forty-eight hours unless you are under medical supervision.

- A two-day water-only fast is the quickest weight-loss method.

- Adequate water intake is a key to healthy fasting.

- A two-week, high-carbohydrate, largely plant-based diet is a safe alternative for those who choose not to fast.

Chapter 4

TAKING IT OFF AND KEEPING IT OFF: DR. STERN'S ROTATION DIET

Dr. Stern's Rotation Diet combines diverse weight-loss plans into a single rotational program of unparalleled effectiveness.

Once you've accomplished the initial fast weight-loss program outlined in the previous chapter it's time to move to a rotational plan that can help you continue toward your weight-loss goals and, once achieved, maintain your chosen weight.

WHAT'S MY CHOSEN WEIGHT?

There's a target weight that will work for you, that will allow you to enjoy life to its fullest, stay in good health, and add years to your lifespan. Your target weight is entirely up to you, but for a general guideline I recommend using a *body mass index*, or *BMI*, chart. They're readily and feely available online (just search for "BMI chart"). Find one and look up your BMI at your current weight (you'll also need to know your height). This will tell you your current BMI. For example, if you are five-foot-eight and 240 pounds, your BMI is 37%; at 175 pounds it's 26%. Then look up your ideal BMI so you know your target healthy weight. Bear in mind that BMI charts are imprecise. Those with a lot of muscle mass, wide hips, or large breasts may need to add a few pounds to what the chart considers a healthy weight. Your goal throughout your dieting should be to maintain a weight within a chosen proximity to your healthy BMI weight. I try to stay within ten pounds and that's what I recommend for you, too. More than a ten-pound range is a little too loose for my tastes, but less than ten pounds might be okay for those who really want to take control and keep a steady course. One more important thing: Your ideal body weight should also make you feel good. If you feel vaguely uncomfortable at your target weight, consider making an adjustment.

Alternatively, if you don't feel that the BMI charts work for you, you can use the height and weight charts included here. They assume that you are between twenty-five and fifty-nine years old, and wearing five pounds of clothing with one-inch heels. Weights are in pounds.

Dr. Stern's Rotation Diet

MEN

| HEIGHT | | WEIGHT | | |
FEET	INCHES	SMALL FRAME	MED. FRAME	LARGE FRAME
5	2	128-134	131-141	138-150
5	3	130-136	133-143	140-153
5	4	132-138	135-145	142-156
5	5	134-140	137-148	144-160
5	6	136-142	139-151	146-164
5	7	138-145	142-154	149-168
5	8	140-148	145-157	152-172
5	9	142-151	148-160	155-176
5	10	144-154	151-163	158-180
5	11	146-157	154-166	161-184
6	0	149-160	157-170	164-188
6	1	152-164	160-174	168-192
6	2	155-168	164-178	172-197
6	3	158-172	167-182	176-202
6	4	162-176	171-187	181-207

| | | WOMEN | | |
| HEIGHT | | WEIGHT | | |
FEET	INCHES	SMALL FRAME	MED. FRAME	LARGE FRAME
4	10	102-111	109-121	118-131
4	11	103-113	111-123	120-134
5	0	104-115	113-126	122-137
5	1	106-118	115-129	125-140
5	2	108-121	118-132	128-143
5	3	111-124	121-135	131-147
5	4	114-127	124-138	134-151
5	5	117-130	127-141	137-155
5	6	120-133	130-144	140-159
5	7	123-136	133-147	143-163
5	8	126-139	136-150	146-167
5	9	129-142	139-153	149-170
5	10	132-145	142-156	152-173
5	11	135-148	145-159	155-176
6	0	138-151	148-162	158-179

WHY DR. STERN'S ROTATION DIET?

Remember, your body is designed to gain weight. Whenever you try to lose weight you are working against everything that your body is designed to do. Maybe evolution will eventually catch up and our bodies will stop trying to make us fat, but it hasn't happened yet and it isn't going to for a long, long time. Here's why: Plentiful food is a new phenomenon. Throughout the majority of human history, food scarcity has been the rule. There was usually less food than we needed, so our bodies learned to store as much as possible for future use. People in ancient societies were rarely fat because most of them could never eat enough to get that way. It was literally impossible. In fact, so few people had unfettered access to food that obesity was often considered a sign of prestige and good health. Here in the Western World, food scarcity persisted right up into the nineteenth century, and even today there are places where it remains the status quo. So as

80

you can see, your body isn't going to rewire itself any time soon, and that may be a good thing. After all, our current age of plenty may be just a blip in the big picture of human history. Either way, one thing's for sure: Keeping off excess fat and maintaining a reasonably trim figure means going to war against your body's basic instincts.

When you put yourself on a weight-loss diet (and I'm talking about a long-term diet, not a short rapid-weight-loss plan like we discussed in the previous chapter), you disrupt your body's norms. Gone are the processed, high-fat foods that you've eaten for years. Now maybe you're sticking to lean high-protein foods. That's great, but here's what's likely to happen next.

Your Body Will Strike Back. Your body's job is to store fat. It does so for your own welfare. Your diet will work, but over time it will become less effective as your body finds ways to circumvent it. It will find the hidden fats that you don't even know you're eating and pack away every molecule. After a while, even with strict adherence, you'll begin to notice that the same things you've been doing successfully aren't working as well as they used to. You might notice your weight creeping back up, and you'll find yourself working harder and harder just to stay in one place.

You Will Get Bored. Boredom is a great scourge of human existence. We spend massive amounts of money keeping ourselves entertained. Sometimes we even put ourselves in debt buying expensive TVs and elaborate vacations, yet we rarely think of *eating* as a source of entertainment. How often do we snack because we're genuinely hungry? Sometimes, sure, but most of the time we're just bored. A bag of Fritos passes the time and engages the senses: It's the very definition of entertainment.

And this points up a problem with many weight-loss diets: Either they're boring to begin with or they become boring over time. Boredom begets cheating, and cheating ruins diets. Remember, all diets work; it's the people who fail.

Dr. Stern's Rotation Diet to the Rescue! Dr. Stern's rotation diet addresses both of these issues to help keep you on track for long-term weight loss and weight maintenance. By the time your body catches on to your dieting schemes you will have moved on to a new one. Just as you start to get bored with what you're doing you'll be ready to move on to something new and exciting. And, of course, there's a lot to be said for always having something to look forward to. Knowing that a change is coming is also a great way to stay energized, engaged, and motivated.

STARTING DR. STERN'S ROTATION DIET

First, if you feel that you need to lose a significant amount of weight, start with the fasting method outlined in the previous chapter. Once your fasting is completed, spend a few days transitioning back to solid foods, first with liquids like consommé and fresh-squeezed juices, on the second day go to more solid foods like Jell-O and raw vegetables, and on the third day add cooked vegetables and rice.

Once you've completed that, it's time to pick three diets that you'd like to try. Revisit *What's Out There and Why You Should Know* a couple chapters back as a general guide, but remember that the example diets that I provided are just that: examples. There are zillions of other diets out there, but virtually all of them will fit into one of my broad categories (low-carb diets, ideological diets, etc.). For your first rotation, here's what I recommend . . .

Start With a Low-Carb Diet: The first time you do this you'll be coming off of your first fast, which transitioned to a meal-replacement diet, which now transitions to a low-carb diet. Replace one of your meal-replacements with a small solid-food meal of egg, meats, and dairy. Don't overdo it; no matter how intensely you may crave it, your body won't be ready for a heavy, solid meal yet. Keep your portion small and modest.

For a week, continue to transition. Decrease meal replacements and increase your new low-carb diet until you have switched entirely to the new diet. Then stick with it for a month, recording your impressions and progress in your journal. When the month is over, it's time to rotate again.

Next, Try a Low-Fat Diet. Again, transition between diets. Spend a week reducing fatty foods while increasing whole grains, beans, and other complex carbohydrates until you are entirely on a low-fat diet. Record your impressions and results in your journal.

WHAT HAVE YOU ACCOMPLISHED?

Here's what: In less than half a year you will have tried four diets: fasting, meal-replacement, low-carb, and low-fat. You will have a good, working knowledge of how each one affects your mind and your body. And if you followed the rules and stuck to the plan, you will have lost weight. You'll understand how to transition from one diet to another, and you'll be ready to try some new diet variations.

WHERE DO WE GO FROM HERE?

As you strike out on your own and you customize your diet rotation to meet your personal needs and goals, remember that the greatest variety and effectiveness comes with picking diets from different categories. If you want to try a diet that's significantly different from any others you've followed, consider taking it for a ten-day test drive. Transition into it, then pay attention, stick to the rules, and don't cheat. Following a diet faithfully and correctly is the only way to gauge its worth. Here's what to look for:

Do You Lose Weight? This is a no-brainer, but it still must be said: Check your weight every day. If your chosen diet is going to work for you, you should experience some weight loss within the ten-day trial period. If you don't, consider scrapping it and trying a different diet.

Can You Tolerate it? Can you imagine living with this diet for a while? Remember, you're bound to like some diets better than others, but if you really can't stand a given diet then you'll find yourself looking for ways to cut corners and cheat. Therefore, I recommend avoiding any diets that you sincerely dislike.

But if your answer to both of the above questions is yes, then you may have found a winner. After a year you'll have a solid understanding of how different types of diets affect you both physically and psychologically, which means you'll have a better knowledge of how food impacts your life than ninety percent of your peers.

Summing it up . . .

- Identify your current BMI and your ideal BMI (or use my alternative chart). Your ideal BMI is your weight-loss goal.

- A long-term weight-loss program disrupts your body's norms and your body will push back.

- Boredom is a major factor in weight-loss failure.

- Dr. Stern's Rotation diet addresses these issues by keeping your body off balance and providing variety.

- Try three diets in rotation, always being careful to transition from one to the other.

- Customize your program to meet your personal tastes and weight-loss goals.

Chapter 5

STAY THE COURSE: THE CHALLENGE OF WEIGHT MAINTENANCE

Why is it so hard to maintain our chosen weight? It's because our bodies and minds conspire against us. Learn how to fight back!

Gaining weight is easy and fun. Losing weight is difficult but do-able, and it's worth the effort and sacrifice. Whether we realize it or not, we are all on a diet; the only question is, which diet are we on? Again, broadly speaking, there are only three kinds:

1. A weight-loss diet (WLD)
2. A weight-neutral (or weight-maintenance) diet (WND)
3. A weight-gaining diet (WGD)

A diet that includes anything you want in any quantity is a *weight-gaining diet*. I've been on that diet and it works, but it's not the diet that I recommend.

When we make the commitment to follow a weight-loss diet we often find that, once our goal is achieved and we think the hard part is behind us, maintaining our chosen weight is almost as hard as losing the weight to begin with. Why is this, and how does Dr. Stern's Rotation Diet help address these issues?

Losing Weight Slows Your Metabolism. Metabolism varies from person to person. We've all met that person who can eat a gallon of ice cream in a single sitting and never gain an ounce. Far more common, sadly, is the person who can't eat a single chocolate-chip cookie without seeing a weight gain. You probably have some idea of how your own metabolism works because you've had to live with it your whole life (don't get too comfortable, because it will probably change as you age), but dieting will throw your metabolism out of whack and confound your expectations. Specifically, it will *slow it down,* making it harder to lose weight and keep it off. Every bite you take will have more weight-gaining potential than it used to, and the fact that you're getting older only makes it worse.

Your metabolism slows down when you lose weight, which means that the more you *lose* weight the easier it is to *gain* weight. Your satiety (or sense of fullness) decreases and your appetite increases due to the hormones *leptin* and *ghrelin*. Leptin is an appetite inhibitor, making you feel full and satisfied; ghrelin is often called the "hunger hormone" because it does the opposite by increasing appetite. Blood levels of ghrelin are highest before meals when hungry, returning to lower levels after meals. Making things even harder is the fact that the more you exercise the more efficient your muscles become at completing the same tasks, therefore burning fewer calories and forcing you to increase or modify your fitness regimen just to keep burning the same number of calories as before.

One way to push back against all of this is by changing your diet. Transitioning the nature of your food intake on a monthly basis can help keep your metabolism off balance. It doesn't give it the opportunity to settle in and get comfortable with your body's "new normal." Also, high-fiber and high-protein foods can boost your metabolism, so every time you switch to a high-fiber or high-protein diet you'll give yourself a metabolism boost that can help your body process more of what you've consumed without converting it to fat.

We Rely too Much on Movement to do the Job for Us. Movement (or exercise) is great and I encourage it. Whether you have a bona fide fitness regimen at the local gym, or just like to take a walk around the block in the evening, movement will improve your mood, enhance your well-being and, yes, burn some calories. For weight maintenance, though, it isn't all it's cracked up to be.

Movement and diet are two different activities that accomplish two different things. A fitness regimen will help keep you fit, just as the name implies, and when done properly it can also be a helpful aid to weight loss. I recommend moderate to vigorous exercise for 150-250 minutes a week focused mostly on aerobic cardiovascular training with a measure of resistance training for toning and increasing muscle mass.

Be aware, though, that intense movement for more than 250 minutes a week may have detrimental effects on weight loss because it will increase your appetite and make it harder for you to restrict your intake.

Do your cardio and your weight training and anything else that helps you keep your heart and lungs healthy and your muscles toned, but remember that movement isn't your primary weapon in the weight-loss battle. That's what your diet is for. Weight maintenance has far more to do with eating than with activity. Keeping your calorie count down is the first line of defense against backsliding on your weight goals. So by all means, do your cardio and keep yourself in shape, but watching what you eat and sticking with Dr. Stern's Rotation Diet will do more to keep you trim than exercise ever will, so limit your intake and stay with the plan.

We Lose Focus and Discipline. When we begin anything—a new job, a marriage, a course of study, a diet—we do so with energy and enthusiasm. But what happens when the novelty wears off, and what used to be new and exciting becomes routine, boring, and even annoying? We slack off, we cut corners at work, we grunt at our spouses, we skip classes, and we gobble up donuts. Sticking to a diet is hard. You'll want to rebel and do all the things you know you're not supposed to do, and you'll probably fall off the wagon once or twice. It happens; don't beat yourself up about it, but do get back on the wagon and carry on. If you make a habit of slipping or, worse, abandon the program entirely, you will lose everything that you've accomplished and end up right where you were when you started: trying to figure out how to lose weight (and maybe telling yourself that Dr. Stern's Rotation Diet didn't work). It will work if you do, and it will work if you stick with it even when you feel like quitting.

WHAT HAPPENS IF I STILL GAIN WEIGHT IN SPITE OF ALL MY EFORTS?

Dr. Stern's Rotation Diet works, but you can't stop your body from aging, changing, and adapting. You certainly shouldn't see any rapid or significant weight gain, but if you do find yourself gradually exceeding the acceptable weight range that you've established for yourself, that's when it's time to go back to square one and do a reset. Start over again with a two-day fast (water only), transition into meal supplements, and then go back to the rotation diet. Weigh yourself every day and track your progress. You'll probably find that your weight stabilizes again and you're back where you want to be.

Weight maintenance demands eternal vigilance. Stay faithful to your diet, make it a priority, track your weight, don't cheat and, most importantly, when you find yourself flagging, remind yourself of why you wanted to lose weight to begin with. Staying in touch with that original impulse is the most powerful force that you can harness to keep yourself on track for the long haul. Motivation is essential, and it's what we'll talk about next.

Summing it up . . .

- There are only three types of diets: weight loss, weight neutral, and weight gaining.

- Weight loss slows your metabolism, making it easier to gain weight. Counteract this by rotating your diet.

- Movement (exercise) alone isn't enough to maintain your weight.

- Loss of focus and discipline will sabotage your efforts.

- Your program will require adjustments as your body changes and ages. Stay in touch with yourself and remain vigilant.

Chapter 6

THE KEY TO SUCCESS: MO-TIVATION

Motivation is the element that separates success from failure. Find your motivation and harness it to reach your goals.

I was once told that there were no known premature deaths from heart disease (the number-one cause of death in the US) among those who had run a marathon. Imagine that: Run a marathon and have one less type of mortality to worry about. It would be like having an insurance policy against early heart disease! All I had to do was run a marathon.

We should all be motivated by the promise of good health, but the evidence that we are not is all around us. Many of us require a little something more to get us going and *keep* us going. There are plenty of things that we could all do to stave off premature heart disease, but most of us don't do them. The real roots of my motivation ran deeper: All three of my mother's siblings and her father had died of heart disease; two of my uncles died very prematurely at forty-five and forty-two years old, respectively. My wife's father also died prematurely of a massive heart attack when she was only fourteen years old. Cardiac health was on my mind.

So I ran the 1978 New York City Marathon and all along the route, through all five boroughs, the crowds shouted my name: *Mickey!* What a rush it was to hear the crowd call out to me, urging me on through every mile toward the distant finish line. Never mind the fact that the guy right behind me wore a bright Mickey Mouse t-shirt. As far as I was concerned, they were shouting for *me!* I finished that marathon and I liked it so much that I ran two more, plus a triathlon. As it turns out, though, I had been misinformed: Marathon runners *do* get heart disease.

Nonetheless, I ran that first marathon because I had found a compelling reason to do so, one that motivated me to plow through the difficult training and conditioning required to run a twenty-six-plus-mile marathon. What motivates *you?*

FOUR IMPORTANT THINGS

As I said at the very beginning of this book, most weight-loss programs have four key components:

- Motivation
- Disciplined Endurance
- Diet
- Exercise

What I didn't say at the beginning of this book is that *motivation* is the most important piece. It's more important than what you eat or how many calories you burn. Without motivation, every diet will fail. In fact, without motivation, very little of what you set out to do in any arena will succeed. To a large extent, your success or failure in any enterprise correlates exactly to your level of motivation.

YOUR COMPELLING WHY

Some people drift through life without direction, rudderless, going wherever the winds take them. They lack purpose. I'm sure you've known a few people like this.

Purpose is what separates doers from drifters. I like to call it your *why,* and it is the first and most important component of motivation. *Why* do you want to lose weight in the first place? The initial spark that ignites your urge may be as vague as a simple desire to lose weight. We're all under pressure from society to look a certain way, thin and in shape. Most of us would like to recapture our nineteen-year-old bodies. Are those reasons enough to keep you going when you're tired of the discipline of dieting and when you're tempted by pizza and cheesecake? They might be. But you might have to dig a little deeper to find what really compels you, to find your *why.* Would you like to see your grandchildren graduate from college? Would you like to meet your great-granddaughter? Or maybe you'd like to regain the mobility and energy that you enjoyed twenty years ago? Weight loss is a great way to recapture some of the feeling of youth and, if you're a guy, having a decent body can help compensate for your receding hairline. There's also the classic *beach-body* inducement, and the *class-reunion* motivation can be powerful, but you'll have to find something else to keep you going after the event is over and your classmates are done trying to remember your name.

The point is that you have to discover what motivates *you*. Find something personal, something that resonates with you, something that makes the work and the sacrifice mean more than a vague desire to lose weight. It might even shift from week to week. What motivates you now may not motivate you next year, but something will. Dig deep, find it, get in touch with it, and make it your cause. Make it your *why*. Do this and, when you are offered pizza and cheesecake, you will simply ask yourself: *Why* am I losing weight? You will remember why. And you will say no to temptation.

ACCENTUATE THE POSITIVE

Human beings seem to be hardwired to think the worst. *I can't do it. I'm not smart enough for this. I'm not attractive enough. I'll never land that job. I can't lose weight.* Even those who seem to have optimistic and sunny dispositions are often wracked with self-doubt.

The truth is that our self-doubts sabotage us and prevent us from doing the things that could create massive improvements in our own lives and in the lives of others. The most insidious thing of all is that our self-doubts are often unconscious. They creep around beneath our thoughts, just out of sight, but we still hear them and they influence everything we do. How can we fight such a stealthy and destructive enemy?

Here's how: Train yourself to recognize negative thoughts. When your hear that voice or feel that nagging doubt, stop it in its tracks and counter it with a positive rejoinder: *I will do it. I am smart enough for this. I am attractive enough. I will get that job. I will lose weight.*

Then take it a step further. It's one thing to harness the unconscious thoughts that whizz through your head and make them do your bidding; it's another to bombard yourself with *conscious* positive thoughts. Make a point to talk to yourself throughout the day, telling yourself that your goals are within your reach and that you have the power to grasp them. You'll be amazed by the lift that this simple technique will have on your spirits, and the brighter your spirits the easier it will be to lose weight. Negative people don't lose weight; positive people do. When you believe you can do it, when you *know* you can do it, you will do it.

If you pray before meals, include this mantra when you do: *The less I eat, the better I feel and the healthier I get.* I can't tell you how many mental battles I won by just saying *Eat less, lose more.*

Decide how to answer others when they ask you how you're doing. It happens every day: Someone says, *How are you?* It isn't so much a question as a standard greeting, but the way you answer it can make an impact on your mood. Choose the most positive word in your vocabulary and make that your answer. I always say *Super!* And every time I say it, it makes me feel that way. It'll work for you, too.

One more thing: Don't get hung up on your sacrifices. It's easy to mourn the things you've given up when you're tempted with pizza and cheesecake. When you feel those pangs of envy and regret, remind yourself of what you gain by giving up those pleasures. You could enjoy the fleeting experience of a bowl of potato chips, or you could enjoy another year of life. When looked at in those terms, it's easy to resist temptation with no regrets and actually feel good about it.

ALWAYS SOMETHING THERE TO REMIND ME

In the same way that your body works against you when you're dieting, your brain will work against you too. Your efforts to motivate yourself and stay positive will be under constant assault from a brain that seeks to undermine you. Why does it do this? No one knows, it's just a bizarre quirk of human nature. But, once again, you can counteract it and triumph. One weapon in your arsenal is the *reminder*. Use Post-It Notes to leave messages with encouraging phrases (*You got this! Stay on target! You can do it!*) wherever you're likely to encounter them: on the bathroom mirror, in your sock drawer, on the dashboard, on your computer monitor, in the refrigerator, you name it. It sounds a little silly, and people might look at you funny, but here's the thing: Successful people all around the world use this method to keep themselves on track. It really works. Leaving yourself positive notes is like launching a full-frontal assault on creeping negativity. And if anyone looks at you funny, just think of how they'll look at you when you're twenty pounds lighter.

PILLOW TALK

When you're asleep, your subconscious mind takes over and has free rein. As much influence as your backwater thoughts have when you're awake, at night they have your head all to themselves and they can do a lot of damage. Fight back by getting into the habit of telling yourself positive affirmations as you fall asleep. Remind yourself of the day's triumphs, express gratitude for opportunities and unexpected gifts, and look forward to the wonderful things that the next day has in store. In the morning, repeat the process. Each time you do this you will set the stage for positive subconscious thoughts at night, and a productive day tomorrow. It's a simple, five-minute routine that guarantees you'll never wake up on the wrong side of the bed again.

IT CAN BE DONE!

When things get you down and you feel like you'll never accomplish your goal, always remember *me*. All of the advice in this book comes from someone who is a quadriplegic unable to walk or roll over or lift weights. If I can do it despite my challenges, you can certainly do it. Feel free to cut out my picture and tape it on the wall as a reminder. Anyone who wants to switch bodies for the day is welcome to mine.

STAY IN TOUCH

Above all, stay in touch with your *why*. That is the most important thing. Just like checking the scale, it's essential to rekindle, every day, the motivation that drives you onward. If you let it cool, your weight-loss goal and all of the benefits that come with it will be in jeopardy. Everything else in this chapter is designed to reinforce your *why*, to keep it effective, to let it do its job to push you toward your goal.

And you *will* reach your goal if you take the advice in this book, but the tips and tricks in *this* chapter will benefit every area of your life. Every obstacle that you face, every challenge that confronts you, every setback that confounds you, can be cut down to size through positivity, motivation, and having a compelling *why*. It will enhance and fortify your entire life. Weight loss is only the beginning.

Summing it up . . .

- **Motivation is the key element that will drive you to success.**
- **Find your compelling *why* and remind yourself of it consistently.**
- **Eliminate negative thinking; reorient pessimism into optimism.**
- **Create a positive mantra and repeat it to yourself throughout the day.**
- **Focus on benefits, not sacrifices.**
- **Find creative ways to remind yourself of positive messages.**
- **Repeat affirmations as you fall asleep.**

Chapter 7

EVERYONE'S LIFELONG STRUGGLE

Weight maintenance is a lifelong commitment. Here are some techniques to help you stay at your desired target.

So you've reached your ideal weight. I wish I could tell you that you can relax, rest on your laurels, and never again worry about what you eat. Alas, I cannot. Maintaining a weight within your ideal range takes constant vigilance and an unending commitment to healthy diets. If that sounds like a drag, fear not. The changes that you make in your diet and habits, based on the advice in this book, create benefits that go far beyond maintaining a healthy weight. You'll enjoy increased energy and sex drive; a clearer mind; reduced risk of cancer, diabetes, and heart disease; better health; and a longer lifespan, just to name a few. What will you give up? Gluttony, junk food, sweets, and undisciplined eating. Sounds like a pretty good deal to me.

Losing weight and *maintaining* weight are two different things. After losing weight, your body burns less energy with exercise, your appetite increases, and your feeling of fullness is reduced. All of this is in addition to a plethora of hormones that work against your effort to maintain your weight, subverting it by trying to store fat instead. The deck is always stacked against you.

In order to maintain your weight after losing it you have to consume approximately 150 calories a day less than your norm, and exercise 200 calories more, just to keep your current weight compared to someone who has been stable at the same weight for years.

So what do you do? After you've used Dr. Stern's Rotation Diet to achieve a weight within your chosen range, based upon your body mass index, it's time to shift gears into maintenance mode.

WHAT'S THE SECRET OF MAINTAINING WEIGHT?

The secret is to lose weight to within a range of your BMI ideal:

- Within 5% if your ideal weight is between 100 and 150 pounds

- Within 7% if your ideal weight is between 150 and 200 pounds

So if your ideal weight is 175 pounds, you are within your range at 187 pounds (stick with the discipline and you'll lose those last twelve pounds, too). If your ideal weight is between 200 and 250 pounds, then you can get within 10% of your ideal weight.

No one under seven feet tall—and that describes most of us—should have an ideal weight that exceeds 250 pounds; if you're under six feet tall, your ideal weight should never be over 200 pounds (Please bear in mind that the guidelines mentioned in this chapter are not exact science and that adjustments may need to be made for heavy musculature and body type).

Weigh yourself every day. If you get within a percent of exceeding your maintenance range, it's time to take action: Go on a two-day water fast or a five-day meal replacement with a program that provides 600 to 800 calories a day. Then return to your regular diet.

Do you have to watch what you eat for the rest of your life? Yes, you do. If you're religious, you have to pray every day for the rest your life. If you want to be physically fit, you can't just exercise for two years and expect to reap the benefits for the rest of your life. It's a lifetime commitment to well-being, happiness, and improved longevity.

Yes, this is hard, but it keeps you within your ideal weight range. It also illustrates the importance of discipline and mindfulness. Check your weight every day and immediately take action when necessary. This is where most people fail, and where you need to focus your attention once you have successfully achieved your weight-loss goal. Failure to do so will put you at risk of further weight gain which will require even stronger measures to control.

THE CASE FOR ONGOING FASTING

I recently made a profound discovery: The more I eat, the more I want to eat. There's a whole category of restaurants based upon this principle: the all-you-can-eat buffet. Strictly in terms of hunger, most of us are satisfied after one serving, and yet we keep going back to the buffet and loading our plates and eating the food. One way to keep this urge in check is to eat less, and one way to eat less is to do a periodic fast. This maintenance option will help enormously with your ongoing commitment to stay within your weight range, and it's pretty simple and straight-forward: On Sunday night, when you go to bed, begin a thirty-six hour water-only fast until you wake up on Tuesday morning (or any other span of days that works with your schedule). If you overeat by 500 calories every day, this weekly fast will erase your excesses. It doesn't give you a license to overeat, but it does give you an es-cape valve. Do a thirty-six-hour fast every week and the risk of exceeding your range will plummet like a stone.

Even better: it provides a way to enjoy large holiday meals without having to endure the associated weight gain. You can enjoy Thanksgiving dinner without guilt if, a day or two later, you embark on a thirty-six-hour fast. It's the best of both worlds, and you'll be thrilled with the freedom and the results.

A VARIATION FOR FASTING-PHOBES

Fasting provides tremendous results, but it's about as pleasant as going thirty-six hours without a bite to eat. I get it. Nonetheless, I still recommend the fast, but if fasting is more than you can bear, I have an easier option: The TRF.

TRF stands for *time-restricted feeding*. Follow the thirty-six-hour fast as outlined above, but make one crucial change: On Monday, at 7:00 p.m., allow yourself one 300-calorie meal.

Otherwise, adhere to the fast. That small meal helps break up the fast, it gives you a waypoint and something to look forward to, and it helps alleviate discomfort.

TWO MORE TOOLS FOR CHRONIC CASES

The word *chronic* gets thrown around a lot in our day-to-day language, so let's be clear about what it really means: *continuing or occurring again and again for a long time* (Thanks to Merriam-Webster for the definition). Chronic weight issues may require stronger tools than a self-administered weight-loss program.

Tool number one is the many board-certified weight-loss physicians in most communities who offer pharmacotherapy or prescription medication that can aid you in your quest to lose weight. Unfortunately, these are not prescribed on a chronic basis despite the fact that obesity is a chronic disease and should be treated as such, utilizing medication when needed for lifelong weight maintenance.

The second tool has the best long-term success rate for significantly overweight patients who seek to lose weight and maintaining it for long periods of time: bariatric surgery, including gastric bypass, performed by board-certified specialists who have access to the latest techniques and procedures.

While these tools are available to you, and should be kept in mind, I recommend starting with Dr. Stern's Rotation Diet. Adopt it as a new and permanent part of your lifestyle and let it do its work. If, in spite of all your efforts, you still can't achieve satisfactory minimum results please consult a board-certified specialist in your area for more help.

IT'S ALL UP TO YOU

Remember that your journey will have peaks and valleys and plateaus. If your weight-loss stalls, that's okay. A pause isn't the same thing as backsliding. Celebrate your progress so far and move on. The work doesn't stop, it just changes.

Don't ease up when you reach your goal, and don't put your hard-won achievements at risk by slacking off after you arrive at your destination. Stick with the program and make the program stick.

Summing it up . . .

- **The secret of maintaining weight is to lose weight to within a percentage of your ideal BMI and work to stay within that range.**

- **A weight-loss diet isn't a once-and-done affair. It's a lifetime commitment.**

- **Periodic fasting can help you stay on target and make up for occasional lapses like holiday meals.**

- **Time-restricted feeding is a kinder and gentler alternative to fasting.**

- **For chronic cases, board-certified physicians can provide medical alternatives, including bariatric surgery and prescription medications, to help you reach your ideal body weight.**

Chapter 8

MINDFULNESS

A simple awareness of what you eat—and of everything else that you do—will profoundly impact your weight-loss journey and every other aspect of your life.

It isn't easy being a virtual quadriplegic. Other than having partial use of one arm, my ability to move my body without assistance is confined to my head and neck. It's a situation that I wouldn't wish on anyone, and I'm not reminding you of it to gain your sympathy. I'm reminding you because it's difficult to imagine being in a more challenging weight-loss and weight-maintenance situation, and yet I have succeeded. Aside from maintaining discipline, keeping my eyes on the prize, staying in touch with my *why*, and taking it seriously, there is one more element of success, one that we touched on earlier, that has helped me succeed: *Mindfulness*.

Mindfulness is a bracingly simple concept with profound implications. On a basic level, it means developing an awareness of the day-to-day habits and activities that we often perform on autopilot. In the context of diet and weight loss, it means being aware of what you eat and the effect that food has on your body, mind, and mood.

You might think, "Of course I'm aware of what I eat!" You probably are. But mindful eating goes beyond simply knowing that there's a piece of roast beef at the end of your fork. It's about true focus and awareness.

Plan your portions ahead of time. If it's a piecemeal food, like french fries, count the pieces. If it's something that isn't easily counted, measure it by volume: teaspoons, tablespoons, cups, etcetera. The point is to decide what you will consume, and how much, before you begin to eat. For example, I might count out a small serving of blueberries, strawberries, and nuts, along with two teaspoons of ice cream. Regardless of what you eat, I recommend limiting your intake to no more than 100 calories at a time. Portion out your food, learn what works for you, and record this information in your journal.

When you sit down to eat, especially if you're alone, make a point to eat slowly and really focus on what you're doing. Think about the flavors, the textures, how the food changes as you chew it, the aftertaste it leaves in your mouth after swallowing. Eating has, all too often, become an afterthought, something we do in the background while socializing, watching TV, or reading. When we make eating an afterthought it becomes mindless, and mindless eating is the gateway to overeating. How many chicken wings does it take to satisfy your hunger? Now ask yourself how many chicken wings you'll eat while you watch a football game. Those are two different—probably *very* different—amounts of chicken wings. Mindful eating will make you understand your ideal portion size. Pay attention to your sensation of hunger as you eat. When you feel satisfied, stop. Think about what you've consumed, and look at what's left on your plate. Adjust your next portion size accordingly.

Focus on your meals. Make your meals the center of mealtime instead of making mealtime a sideshow. You will eat less and you will enjoy it more. After you've eaten, shift your mindfulness to how you feel afterward. Different foods will affect you differently. How do you feel after eating a salad? A stir fry? A steak? A McDonald's Quarter Pounder? A bowl of ice cream? A bowl of rice? A bag of potato chips? Some foods will energize you, others will make you sluggish. Some will almost put you to sleep.

Furthermore, what you eat affects your mind. How's your mood after any given meal? How's your thinking? Is it crisp and clear, or are your thoughts muddled? If all you feel like doing after a meal is sitting on the couch and watching TV it might be time to rethink your diet. Make a note of these things in your journal and take them into account as you plan your meals.

As I said above, mindful eating also has the effect of making you more aware of your ideal portion size. You'll gradually come to understand the volume of food that it takes to satisfy you, and it's probably less—maybe a *lot* less—than you're used to. You'll soon find yourself marveling at the colossal size of restaurant portions and you'll say to yourself, *How could I have ever eaten so much?*

Your diet affects so much more than your weight. It impacts virtually every aspect of your being. Mindful eating will help you refine your diet, control your weight, and improve your mood. Even better: Practicing mindfulness in one area of your life has a positive spillover effect on all other areas. You'll find yourself more aware of everything going on around you. More aware-ness means more opportunities to control your environment, and the more you can control your environment the better off you'll be. And that's a dieting side effect we can all look forward to.

Summing it up . . .

- **Mindfulness means developing an awareness of the day-to-day habits and activities that we often perform on auto-pilot.**

- **In the context of diet and weight loss, mindfulness means being aware of what you eat and the effect that food has on your body, mind, and mood.**

- **Plan portions ahead of time. Carefully measure or count each food.**

- **Focus on the sensations and process of each and every bite.**

- **Make meals the center of mealtime instead of making mealtime a sideshow.**

Chapter 9

MEDITATION

Meditation clears away mental clutter and brings the entire force of your mind to bear on whatever you choose to focus on.

You've probably noticed that this book contains some things that you might not associate with weight-loss books, things like chapters on motivation and mindfulness. Here's another one, and it also begins with M: *Meditation.*

It's become abundantly clear to me over the years that the psychological aspect of weight loss is more important than the dietary and fitness aspects. In fact, your success hinges on it. One of the surest ways to make the psychological aspects stick, to reinforce your efforts, and to shore up your gains, is to bring the power of meditation to bear on your quest.

WHY MEDITATE?

Our days are filled with mental clutter; we're reciting to-do lists and fretting over the day's worries before we even sit down to breakfast. Meditation clears your mind and centers your thoughts. It exerts a calming influence. It resets your brain and makes it receptive to your suggestions (so keep it positive!). Within the context of weight loss, meditation can help you keep it a priority in your daily life when so many other things vie for your attention. It's a time to focus deeply on your *why*. And, like motivation and mindfulness, meditation will improve *every* aspect of your life.

HOW TO DO IT

Meditation can be done at any time of the day or night, but two times you should be *sure* to meditate are shortly after awakening to prepare yourself for the day ahead, and right before bedtime to guide your sleeping subconscious thoughts.

Find a comfortable spot where you can relax. It could be your bed, the floor, the couch, or even the passenger seat of your car (Don't do it while driving!). You can sit or recline, whichever you prefer. Close your eyes. Concentrate on your breathing. Inhale deeply through your nose. Feel your stomach rise with your diaphragm. Hold the breath for a moment. Then exhale slowly through your mouth and feel your abdomen go down. Repeat this ten times while thinking about your ideal location, your ideal temperature, your ideal environment. It could be a beach with rolling surf, a mountain meadow, someplace that you've visited in the past, anyplace that allows you to feel happy, peaceful and content. Make this your personal mental sanctuary and go to it whenever you feel stressed or down. If your mind is troubled, "invite" someone into your sanctuary to share your thoughts. It can be Abraham Lincoln, the Buddha, Jesus Christ, anyone living or dead who appeals to you and brings you understanding, peace, and comfort.

As you continue the breathing exercise, focus on relaxing your body's muscles, one at a time, from head to toe. As you feel the tension drain away and your cares vanish, repeat your personal goals and the reason you want to achieve them. Repeat your *why*. And don't restrict it to weight loss. Whatever you wish to achieve, short term, long term, include them in your meditation. Make your goals and your *why* your personal mantra, unique to you alone.

After repeating the meditation ten times slowly open your eyes, rise to your feet, and proceed with your day (or your slumbers if it's bedtime). Make this the first thing you do every day and the last thing you do at night. Do it as many times as your schedule allows during the day. Do it at lunchtime, do it in the car before driving home in the evening, do it in the shower. You can even do it at the office without leaving your desk. It will make a huge difference in the quality of your life and it will help keep you focused on your weight-loss goals and the *why* that compels you to pursue them.

POSITIVE Q&A

Think of five questions you can ask your-self that have positive, mood-enhancing, life-af-firming answers. Where is the most beautiful place I've ever been? Who loves me more than anyone else? Where is the place that I was happi-est? What is the most successful thing I've ever done? Come up with your own list of five ques-tions and answers, then ask and answer them at least twice a day, in the morning and in the even-ing. It'll give you an instant lift as your day be-gins and as it winds down.

Meditation is a big field and there's more than one way to do it. The methods that I describe here work for me, but I encourage you to try oth-ers. The bottom line is to do it and to make it part of your daily routine. The results will speak for themselves.

Stop for a moment, reread this chapter, and try a meditation exercise before continuing. Do it now while it's fresh in your mind. Concentrate on your breathing; listen to your heartbeat. Take fifteen minutes and enjoy the benefits of meditation.

Summing it up . . .

- **Meditation resets your brain and makes it receptive to your suggestions.**

- **Like motivation and mindfulness, meditation will improve every aspect of your life.**

- **Meditation can be done at any time, but at minimum be sure to do it first thing after awakening and last thing before sleeping.**

- **Find a peaceful place for your meditation and invite people into your mental "sanctuary."**

- **Ask yourself positive questions to reinforce your mood and motivation.**

141

DR. STERN'S HACKS FOR SUCCESSFUL WEIGHT LOSS

A few small hints to help you along your journey to maximum weight loss . . .

Bank Half of Your Meal: Restaurant portions are notoriously large. When you go out to eat, ask the server to put half of your meal in a to-go box *before* it's served. You'll eat half as much, and you'll have another meal to eat later. It's almost like getting two meals for the price of one!

Shrink Your Dishes: Use a half-sized plate, like you might use for bread, for your dinner plate. It'll hold everything you need, and none of what you don't.

Use Cups Instead of Bowls: Whether it's for ice cream, cereal, or soup, a cup holds plenty.

Don't Eat With Your Fingers: Whether it's shoving pizza in your mouth or wolfing down handfuls of peanuts, you will eat more when you eat with your hands. Always use utensils, even with pizza, chips, nuts, and other things that you traditionally eat with your fingers. You'll be more mindful of what you eat and you'll have greater control of the portions. Plus, it's great fun trying to eat potato chips with a fork.

Go OCD on the Finger Foods: When eating finger foods (which you'll eat with utensils), count the number of items and put them in a container before eating. Whether it's grapes, nuts, chips, or any other small pieces, counting them into containers will, again, help you be more mindful of what you eat and will help you control portions.

Guzzle: Drink at least eight ounces of water before eating anything. In addition to keeping you properly hydrated, the water will reduce the space in your stomach and, in turn, reduce your food consumption.

Chew, Don't Swallow: This is a last-resort technique if you fear you're about to fall off of the wagon: If you really can't resist that piece of cake or those potato chips, try chewing without swallowing. I know it's a little gross (Don't do it in a restaurant!), but think about it: Which part of eating generates the most enjoyment? It's the chewing and the tasting. Swallowing is the least of it. So enjoy the cake and the chips without ingesting them. And if you feel that this is a waste of food, remember this: If you spit it out it gets returned to the environment just as much as it does if you swallow it. The net result is the same.

Plan Ahead: Determine the quantities that you'll eat before you sit down to a meal. Portion your food and stick to your decision.

One Size Does Not Fit All: Resign from the clean-plate club. And don't let food companies determine your portions. Just because something is already portioned out doesn't mean you have to abide by their decision. That premade hamburger patty might be twice as much food as you need.

CONCLUSION

Weight loss is hard. It's harder when you're quadriplegic. Maintaining a calorie deficit is seemingly impossible when you spend most of your time strapped to a chair. The calorie-burning day-to-day activities that most people enjoy—walking around, opening jars, bending and stretching, and all the other forms of movement that expends the energy our bodies store—simply don't apply to me. I can move my head and neck and I have limited movement in one arm, so Zumba classes and spin sessions are out of the question.

I'm lucky and grateful to be alive, and my success proves that weight loss and weight maintenance are possible even under the most difficult circumstances. It would be easy for me to make excuses. I could legitimately make just about every one in the book. Instead, I embrace the challenge, make the sacrifices, do the work, and find success.

And it's a good thing I do because, for me, weight loss isn't a luxury. With my health compromised in a number of ways, not to mention the fact that I'm a card-carrying senior citizen, keeping my weight under control is an absolute necessity. In my condition, too much weight would aggravate other issues and reduce both the quantity and quality of my remaining years. It would likely kill me. I will not allow that to happen.

Neither should you. Obesity shortens your life. It's an existential threat. I know it all seems abstract and impossibly far in the future when you're young—it was the last thing on my mind when I was driving through Chicago in my Pontiac Bonneville in the sixties—but believe me when I say that old age doesn't creep up on you. It pounces like a tiger. And suddenly the existential threat of obesity doesn't seem so abstract. Extra weight will rob years from your life and you'll miss them when they're gone, so take control now. It's easier to do it when you're young, when your body still follows orders somewhat. Later in life, your body will become downright rebellious.

While it's important to recognize the threat that obesity poses as we age, that's not how I want to end this book. I want to end it by telling you that the fact that I can lose and maintain weight is proof positive that *anyone* can lose and maintain weight. Your quality of life will improve enormously. You will feel better, think better, and look better. The old cliché was never more true: *You'll add years to your life and life to your years.* It's a good deal, and you'll also reap the benefits of discipline, mindfulness, and meditation, skills that will improve and enhance every facet of your life. The only things that stand in your way are inertia, bad habits, unhealthy eating, and a lack of motivation. There's nothing in that list that can't be overcome if you put your mind to it. You know why it's important. You know how to do it. You know where to go when you need help. Contact me, Dr. Michael Stern, at the Seattle Weight Loss Center for the latest advice, scholarship, and personalized programs to help you achieve your goals.

Establish your goals and get in touch with your *why*. Then, as long as you do your part, Dr. Stern's Rotation Diet will do the rest. I wish you the best of health and success.

And to that I can only add the following: Go forth, take charge, and lose weight!

WHEN YOU NEED MORE HELP

There are a variety of medications available to help you make lifestyle changes and modify your energy intake, and there are dietitians, psychologist, social workers, and physical therapists who can help you with these challenges.

Board-certified physicians specializing in medical treatment of obesity and weight loss can prescribe a variety of medications that will help you reach your individual ideal body weight.

There are also more powerful options that may help. A board-certified obesity physician to get the latest information on the newest drug therapies and surgical procedures that may be recommended for you.

Visit www.SeattleWeightLossCenter.org for the latest information on practitioners in your local area who can help you reach your goals via telemedicine and standard in-office treatments.

ACKNOWLEDGEMENTS

I want to thank all of my friends and family and my caregivers for their support throughout this process.

My sister, Shellie, and my significant other, Viveca, have been instrumental in my completing this book.

The faculty of the obesity seminar of Columbia University who did the basic science research that supports many of my personal beliefs, and all the doctors that have come before who shared their experience on losing and maintaining body weight.

I stand on the shoulders of giants

153

ABOUT DR. MICHAEL STERN

Born and raised on the north side of Chicago, Dr. Michael Stern now resides in Seattle where he is the founder and CEO of the Seattle Weight Loss Center.

Dr. Stern received a Bachelor of Science degree from the University of Wisconsin-Madison, and his MD from the Autonomous University of Guadalajara School of Medicine. He completed six years of residency in internal medicine and general surgery, specializing in adult and pediatric urology and urologic surgery at College of Medicine and Dentistry of New Jersey (now Rutgers New Jersey Medical School), becoming board certified in urology.

Since 1980 Dr. Stern has practiced urology, been an adjunct faculty member at Bastyr University School of Naturopathic Medicine, and taught lifestyle medicine weight loss to his patients. In 2020 he founded the Seattle Weight Loss Center, a nonprofit organization dedicated to helping patients to lose weight fast and forever.

In 1995, Dr. Stern was diagnosed with multiple sclerosis, ending his many athletic pursuits and eventually confining him to a wheelchair as a virtual quadriplegic. In spite of this limitation, and perhaps inspired by it, he has dedicated his life to helping others on their journey towards their bodyweight goals.

Made in USA - Kendallville, IN
1215508_9780578816906
12.17.2020 0856